THE GASTROPARESIS DIET BIBLE

Beginners Guide To Eating Well With Gastroparesis & Tips, Recipes, And Meal Plans

CRUE GAGE

Copyright © 2024 By Crue Gage

All Rights Reserved.

Table of Contents

Introductory 4

CHAPTER ONE 6
   Causes And Symptoms 6
   How Gastroparesis Affects Digestion 9
   Medications For Gastroparesis & Surgical Options 13

CHAPTER TWO 22
   Meal Planning Strategies 22
   Foods To Include In A Gastroparesis Diet 27
   Foods To Avoid With Gastroparesis 33

CHAPTER THREE 38
   7 Days Sample Meal Plans 38
   Breakfast Recipes 48
   Lunch Recipes 53
   Dinner Recipes 59
   Snacks & Desserts Recipes 65

CHAPTER FOUR 72
   Coping With Gastroparesis Symptoms 72
   Conclusion 77

THE END 80

Introductory

Gastroparesis is a condition that results in the delayed evacuation of food from the stomach into the small intestine due to the effects of it on the stomach muscles and nerves. Typically, the stomach contracts to facilitate the passage of food into the small intestine for digestion. However, in gastroparesis, these contractions are impaired or slowed down, resulting in a prolonged period of food retention in the stomach when compared to the norm.

Some common symptoms of gastroparesis include:

- **Nausea and vomiting:** Particularly after eating meals.
- **Feeling full quickly:** Even after consuming small amounts of food.

- **Abdominal bloating:** Due to delayed digestion.
- **Heartburn or gastroesophageal reflux:** When stomach contents back up into the esophagus.
- **Changes in blood sugar levels:** Particularly in individuals with diabetes.

The causes of gastroparesis can vary and may include diabetes, surgery on the stomach or vagus nerve, certain medications, or conditions that affect nerves, such as Parkinson's disease or multiple sclerosis. Treatment options often focus on managing symptoms through dietary changes, medications to stimulate stomach contractions, or in severe cases, surgical interventions.

CHAPTER ONE
Causes And Symptoms

Gastroparesis can be caused by several factors, including:

• **Diabetes:** This is the most common cause of gastroparesis. High blood sugar levels associated with diabetes can damage the vagus nerve, which controls the stomach muscles.

• **Surgery:** Operations on the stomach or upper small intestine can sometimes damage the vagus nerve or the stomach muscles, leading to gastroparesis.

• **Viral infections:** Certain viruses can affect the stomach nerves and cause gastroparesis.

- **Medications:** Some medications, such as opioids and certain antidepressants, can interfere with stomach emptying.

- **Nervous system diseases:** Conditions such as Parkinson's disease, multiple sclerosis, or amyloidosis can affect nerves, including those that control the stomach.

- **Hormonal disorders:** Hypothyroidism (underactive thyroid) and other metabolic disorders can contribute to gastroparesis.

Symptoms of gastroparesis often include:

- **Nausea and vomiting:** Especially after eating.

- **Feeling full quickly:** Even after consuming small amounts of food.

- **Abdominal bloating:** Due to delayed digestion.

- **Heartburn or gastroesophageal reflux:** When stomach contents back up into the esophagus.

- **Changes in blood sugar levels:** Particularly in individuals with diabetes, due to unpredictable digestion times.

Managing gastroparesis typically involves dietary adjustments, medications to help stimulate stomach contractions, managing blood sugar levels (if diabetes-related), and in severe cases, surgical interventions may be considered.

Treatment aims to alleviate symptoms and improve quality of life for individuals with this condition.

How Gastroparesis Affects Digestion

Gastroparesis significantly affects digestion by slowing down or impairing the movement of food through the stomach and into the small intestine. Here's how it impacts digestion:

• **Delayed Gastric Emptying:** The primary issue in gastroparesis is that the stomach muscles don't contract properly or are paralyzed, which delays the passage of food from the stomach into the small intestine. This delay can vary in severity, leading to inconsistent digestion times.

• **Symptoms of Gastroparesis:** Due to delayed gastric emptying, individuals with gastroparesis often experience symptoms such as:

- **Nausea and Vomiting:** Food that remains in the stomach can cause feelings of nausea and may lead to vomiting, especially after meals.

- **Feeling Full Quickly:** Even after consuming small amounts of food, there can be a sensation of fullness and discomfort.

- **Abdominal Pain and Bloating:** The prolonged presence of food in the stomach can cause discomfort, bloating, and pain in the abdominal area.

- **Heartburn and Acid Reflux:** Stomach contents may back up into the esophagus, causing heartburn and discomfort.

- **Malnutrition:** Prolonged gastroparesis can lead to nutritional deficiencies due to impaired absorption of nutrients from food.

- **Impact on Blood Sugar Levels:** For individuals with diabetes, gastroparesis can make it challenging to manage blood sugar levels because food is not digested and absorbed predictably. This can lead to fluctuations in blood glucose levels, making diabetes management more complex.

- **Treatment Approaches:** Managing gastroparesis typically involves dietary adjustments (such as consuming smaller, more frequent meals), medications to stimulate stomach contractions, controlling symptoms like nausea and vomiting, and managing underlying conditions like diabetes. In severe cases, surgical interventions or implantable devices that stimulate stomach muscles may be considered.

Gastroparesis disrupts the normal process of digestion and can significantly impact a person's quality of life, requiring careful management and treatment to alleviate symptoms and prevent complications.

Medications For Gastroparesis & Surgical Options

For gastroparesis, treatment options include both medications and, in some cases, surgical interventions. Here's an overview of each:

Medications for Gastroparesis:

• **Prokinetic Agents:** These medications help stimulate contractions of the stomach muscles, facilitating gastric emptying. Examples include:

• **Metoclopramide:** It enhances stomach contractions and helps reduce nausea and vomiting.

• **Domperidone:** Similar to metoclopramide but with fewer central nervous system side effects; it's not available in all countries.

- **Erythromycin:** Besides being an antibiotic, erythromycin can stimulate stomach contractions and is sometimes used off-label for gastroparesis.

- **Anti-emetics:** These medications help control nausea and vomiting associated with gastroparesis. Examples include:

- **Ondansetron:** Often used to prevent nausea and vomiting.

- **Promethazine or prochlorperazine:** These can also be used to relieve symptoms.

- **Other Medications:** Sometimes medications that affect blood sugar levels (for diabetic gastroparesis) or pain medications may be prescribed depending on individual symptoms and needs.

Surgical Options for Gastroparesis:

• **Gastric Electrical Stimulation (GES):** This involves implanting a device similar to a pacemaker in the abdomen. The device delivers electrical pulses to the stomach muscles, helping to regulate gastric contractions and improve stomach emptying.

• **Gastric Surgery:** In some cases, surgical procedures may be considered to help improve symptoms of gastroparesis. This can include procedures to create a bypass around the stomach (like a gastrojejunostomy) or procedures to help reduce symptoms and improve stomach emptying.

• **Enteral Feeding:** For severe cases where oral intake is severely compromised, feeding tubes may be placed directly into the small intestine to ensure adequate nutrition.

<u>Lifestyle and Dietary Management:</u>

In addition to medications and surgical options, managing gastroparesis often involves dietary modifications such as eating smaller, more frequent meals, avoiding fibrous or high-fat foods, and maintaining adequate hydration. Managing stress levels and staying physically active can also help manage symptoms.

Treatment for gastroparesis is often tailored to the severity of symptoms, underlying causes (like diabetes), and individual responses to various therapies. It's important for individuals with gastroparesis to work closely with healthcare providers to develop a comprehensive treatment plan that addresses their specific needs and improves their quality of life.

Diet plays a crucial role in managing symptoms and meeting nutritional requirements for individuals with gastroparesis. Here's why it's important and how it can help:

Managing Symptoms:

- **Easing Digestion:** Certain foods can aggravate symptoms of gastroparesis, such as nausea, bloating, and abdominal pain. A diet tailored to gastroparesis typically involves consuming smaller, more frequent meals throughout the day. This helps to reduce the amount of food in the stomach at any given time, making digestion easier.

- **Choosing Foods Wisely:** Foods that are easier to digest and pass through the stomach more quickly are often recommended. This includes low-fiber foods (as fiber can be harder to digest), lean proteins, cooked vegetables (which are softer), and easily digestible carbohydrates.

- **Avoiding Trigger Foods:** Some foods can worsen symptoms, such as fatty or fried foods, high-fiber foods (like raw vegetables and whole grains), carbonated beverages, and alcohol. These should be limited or avoided depending on individual tolerance.

Meeting Nutritional Requirements:

- **Preventing Malnutrition:** Gastroparesis can impair the absorption of nutrients from food, leading to potential deficiencies. A balanced diet that focuses on nutrient-dense foods helps ensure adequate intake of essential vitamins, minerals, and proteins.

• **Monitoring Blood Sugar Levels:** For individuals with diabetic gastroparesis, managing carbohydrate intake and monitoring blood sugar levels are crucial. Smaller, more frequent meals that include balanced portions of carbohydrates, proteins, and fats can help stabilize blood sugar levels.

• **Supplementation:** In some cases, dietary supplements may be recommended to help meet nutritional needs, especially if there are concerns about nutrient absorption. This may include vitamin B12, iron, or calcium supplements.

Practical Tips for Dietary Management:

- **Small, Frequent Meals:** Eating smaller portions more frequently throughout the day helps manage symptoms of gastroparesis and aids in digestion.

- **Chewing Thoroughly:** Properly chewing food can ease the workload on the stomach and facilitate digestion.

- **Liquid Foods:** Soups, smoothies, and pureed foods can be easier to digest and may be better tolerated.

- **Hydration:** Maintaining adequate hydration is important, as dehydration can worsen symptoms.

It's beneficial for individuals with gastroparesis to work with a registered dietitian who can develop a personalized meal plan based on their specific needs, symptoms, and nutritional goals. Dietitians can provide guidance on food choices, meal timing, portion sizes, and strategies to manage symptoms effectively.

By focusing on a well-balanced and carefully planned diet, individuals with gastroparesis can better manage their symptoms, support their nutritional needs, and improve their overall quality of life.

CHAPTER TWO
Meal Planning Strategies

Meal planning for gastroparesis involves careful consideration of foods that are easier to digest and less likely to exacerbate symptoms like nausea, bloating, and discomfort. Here are some strategies to help with meal planning:

• Aim to eat smaller meals more frequently throughout the day, rather than three large meals. This helps reduce the volume of food in the stomach at any one time, making digestion easier.

• Choose foods that are soft, tender, and well-cooked. These are generally easier to digest. Examples include steamed vegetables, tender meats, and cooked grains like rice or oatmeal.

- Opt for low-fat foods as fats can slow down digestion. Avoid greasy or fried foods. Limit high-fiber foods such as raw fruits and vegetables, whole grains, and legumes, as these can be harder to digest and may worsen symptoms.

- Include a balance of carbohydrates, proteins, and healthy fats in each meal to help maintain energy levels and support overall health.

- Stay hydrated by sipping fluids throughout the day. Avoid large amounts of liquid at once, as this can also contribute to feelings of fullness and discomfort.

- Choose foods that are easy to chew thoroughly or that are already pureed or mashed. This reduces the workload on the stomach during digestion.

- Identify and avoid foods that trigger symptoms. Common triggers include spicy foods, caffeine, carbonated beverages, alcohol, and high-fat or high-fiber foods.

- Pay attention to portion sizes. Even with smaller meals, overeating can lead to discomfort and worsen symptoms.

Example Meal Ideas:

Breakfast:

- Oatmeal with mashed banana and a small amount of honey.
- Scrambled eggs with well-cooked vegetables.
- Smoothie made with yogurt, banana, and a small amount of spinach.

Lunch:

- Chicken or turkey sandwich on soft bread with lettuce and a small amount of mayonnaise.
- Quinoa salad with soft-cooked vegetables and grilled chicken.
- Soup such as chicken noodle or tomato bisque.

Dinner:

- Baked or grilled fish with steamed carrots and mashed potatoes.
- Pasta with a light tomato sauce and ground turkey.
- Stir-fried tofu with well-cooked vegetables and rice.

<u>Tips for Implementation:</u>

• **Plan Ahead:** Plan meals and snacks in advance to ensure you have suitable options on hand.

- **Listen to Your Body:** Pay attention to how different foods make you feel and adjust your choices accordingly.

By adopting these meal planning strategies, individuals with gastroparesis can help alleviate symptoms, improve digestion, and maintain adequate nutrition for overall health and well-being.

Foods To Include In A Gastroparesis Diet

When planning a diet for gastroparesis, it's important to choose foods that are easy to digest and less likely to exacerbate symptoms like nausea, bloating, and discomfort. Here are some foods that are generally well-tolerated and can be included in a gastroparesis diet:

1. Low-Fat Proteins:

- **Lean meats:** Such as chicken, turkey, fish, and lean cuts of beef or pork.
- **Eggs:** Scrambled or poached eggs are often well-tolerated.
- **Tofu:** Soft or silken tofu can be a good source of protein.

2. Cooked or Soft Vegetables:

- **Root vegetables:** Such as carrots, potatoes (without skin), and sweet potatoes.
- **Well-cooked greens:** Spinach, kale, or Swiss chard, cooked until soft.
- **Zucchini and squash:** These can be steamed or sautéed until tender.

3. Ripe Fruits:

- **Bananas:** Especially ripe bananas, which are easier to digest.
- **Canned fruits:** Like peaches or pears in their own juice (avoid those in heavy syrup).
- **Applesauce:** Unsweetened applesauce can be easier to tolerate than whole apples.

4. Grains and Starches:

- **White rice:** Plain white rice is gentle on the stomach.
- **Pasta:** Choose softer pasta types like macaroni or spaghetti.
- **Oatmeal:** Plain or lightly sweetened oatmeal can be soothing.

5. Dairy and Alternatives:

- **Low-fat or non-fat dairy:** Such as yogurt, milk, or cheese (in moderation).
- **Plant-based milks:** Like almond milk or rice milk, if tolerated.

6. Soups and Broths:

- **Clear broths:** Chicken or vegetable broth can be soothing and hydrating.

- **Pureed soups:** Soups made from well-cooked vegetables, pureed for smoother texture.

7. Soft Breads and Grains:

- **White bread:** Choose softer varieties without seeds or whole grains.
- **Bagels or English muffins:** Plain varieties can be easier to digest.

8. Healthy Fats in Moderation:

- **Avocado:** Mashed or sliced avocado can provide healthy fats.
- **Olive oil:** Use in moderation for cooking or as a dressing.

Tips for Preparation and Consumption:

- **Cooking Methods:** Choose methods like steaming, boiling,

baking, or poaching, which make foods softer and easier to digest.
- **Smaller Portions:** Eat smaller meals more frequently throughout the day to avoid overwhelming the stomach.
- **Chewing Thoroughly:** Properly chew food to aid digestion and reduce the workload on the stomach.
- **Hydration:** Stay hydrated by sipping water or other fluids throughout the day, but avoid large amounts at once.

It's important to note that individual tolerance to foods may vary. Some people with gastroparesis may find certain foods on this list still trigger symptoms. Keeping a food diary can help identify specific triggers and tailor the diet accordingly.

For personalized guidance, especially in managing a gastroparesis diet, consulting with a registered dietitian who specializes in gastrointestinal disorders can be highly beneficial.

They can help create a customized meal plan that meets nutritional needs while managing symptoms effectively.

Foods To Avoid With Gastroparesis

When managing gastroparesis, it's important to avoid foods that can exacerbate symptoms and make digestion more difficult. Here are some common foods and dietary choices that individuals with gastroparesis are often advised to avoid:

1. High-Fat Foods:

- **Fried foods:** French fries, fried chicken, etc.
- **Fatty cuts of meat:** Such as bacon, sausage, and fatty steaks.
- **Creamy sauces:** Heavy cream sauces or gravies.

2. High-Fiber Foods:

- **Whole grains:** Whole wheat bread, whole grain cereals, and brown rice.
- **Raw vegetables:** Raw carrots, broccoli, celery, etc.
- **Legumes:** Beans, lentils, and chickpeas.

3. Tough or Fibrous Meats:

- **Tough cuts of meat:** Such as steak or pork chops.
- **Processed meats:** Hot dogs, sausages, and deli meats.

4. Gas-Producing Foods:

- **Carbonated beverages:** Soda, sparkling water, etc.
- **Cruciferous vegetables:** Cabbage, cauliflower, Brussels sprouts, etc.

5. Spicy or Acidic Foods:

- **Spicy foods:** Hot peppers, chili, curry, etc.
- **Citrus fruits:** Oranges, grapefruits, lemons, etc.

6. Alcohol and Caffeine:

- **Alcoholic beverages:** Beer, wine, spirits.
- **Caffeinated beverages:** Coffee, tea, energy drinks.

7. Large Meals:

- Eating large meals can overwhelm the stomach and exacerbate symptoms. Instead, opt for smaller, more frequent meals throughout the day.

8. Hard or Sticky Foods:

- **Nuts and seeds:** Whole nuts, nut butters with chunks, etc.
- **Chewy candies or snacks:** Caramels, taffy, etc.

Tips for Managing Diet:

- **Keep a Food Diary:** Recording what you eat and how you feel afterward can help identify specific triggers and adjust your diet accordingly.
- **Choose Easy-to-Digest Foods:** Opt for foods that are soft, well-cooked, and easily chewed to reduce the workload on the stomach.
- **Stay Hydrated:** Drink fluids throughout the day, but avoid large quantities at once to prevent further discomfort.

- **Consult a Dietitian:** For personalized advice, especially in managing a gastroparesis diet, working with a registered dietitian who specializes in gastrointestinal disorders can provide valuable guidance.

By avoiding these problematic foods and making thoughtful dietary choices, individuals with gastroparesis can better manage their symptoms and improve their overall quality of life.

CHAPTER THREE
7 Days Sample Meal Plans

Creating a sample meal plan for gastroparesis involves choosing foods that are gentle on the stomach, easy to digest, and less likely to exacerbate symptoms like nausea, bloating, and discomfort. Here's a 7-day sample meal plan to provide some ideas:

Day 1

Breakfast:

- Scrambled eggs with soft-cooked spinach
- White toast (lightly toasted)
- Banana slices

Lunch:

- Chicken and rice soup (pureed for smoother texture)

- Saltine crackers

Dinner:

- Baked salmon with lemon and dill
- Mashed potatoes (without skins)
- Steamed carrots

Snack:

- Applesauce

Day 2

Breakfast:

- Oatmeal with mashed banana and a sprinkle of cinnamon
- Soft-cooked scrambled eggs

Lunch:

- Quinoa salad with cooked vegetables (like zucchini and bell peppers)

- Light vinaigrette dressing

Dinner:

- Turkey meatballs in marinara sauce (pureed or very finely chopped)
- Soft-cooked pasta (like penne or fusilli)

Snack:

- Greek yogurt with honey

<u>**Day 3**</u>

Breakfast:

- Smoothie with yogurt, strawberries, and a tablespoon of almond butter
- Toasted white bread (lightly toasted)

Lunch:

- Chicken salad made with shredded chicken, mayonnaise, and chopped celery (mashed or pureed if needed)
- Soft bread or crackers

Dinner:

- Soft tofu stir-fry with well-cooked vegetables (like carrots, snow peas, and mushrooms)
- White rice

Snack:

- Cottage cheese with canned peaches (in juice, not syrup)

Day 4

Breakfast:

- Scrambled eggs with mashed avocado
- White toast (lightly toasted)

Lunch:

- Tomato soup (smooth and not too thick)
- Saltine crackers

Dinner:

- Baked chicken breast with a light lemon sauce
- Mashed sweet potatoes

Snack:

- Smoothie with yogurt, blueberries, and a teaspoon of honey

Day 5

Breakfast:

- Oatmeal with applesauce and a sprinkle of ground flaxseed
- Soft-cooked scrambled eggs

Lunch:

- Spinach and feta cheese omelet (cooked until very soft)
- Toasted white bread (lightly toasted)

Dinner:

- Grilled fish fillet with a side of steamed broccoli and cauliflower (soft-cooked)

Snack:

- Rice pudding made with almond milk and cinnamon

Day 6

Breakfast:

- Smoothie with banana, spinach, and yogurt
- Soft-cooked scrambled eggs

Lunch:

- Chicken and vegetable broth soup (strained if needed)
- Saltine crackers

Dinner:

- Turkey burger on a soft bun with lettuce and tomato
- Mashed potatoes (without skins)

Snack:

- Applesauce with a sprinkle of cinnamon

Day 7

Breakfast:

- Cottage cheese with canned pears (in juice, not syrup)
- Toasted white bread (lightly toasted)

Lunch:

- Tuna salad made with mashed avocado instead of mayonnaise (soft and easy to chew)
- Soft bread or crackers

Dinner:

- Beef stew (cooked until meat and vegetables are very tender)
- Soft-cooked noodles

Snack:

- Smoothie with yogurt, strawberries, and a tablespoon of almond butter
- Tips for Adapting the Meal Plan:

Adjust portion sizes according to individual tolerance and energy needs. Stay hydrated throughout the day by sipping water or herbal teas between meals. Keep track of how different foods make you feel and adjust your diet accordingly.

This sample meal plan provides a variety of options that are generally well-tolerated by individuals with gastroparesis. It's important to tailor the plan to your own preferences and dietary tolerances while ensuring that you're meeting your nutritional needs.

Breakfast Recipes

Here are a few breakfast recipes that are gentle on the stomach and suitable for individuals with gastroparesis:

1. Simple Scrambled Eggs

Ingredients:

- 2 eggs
- Salt and pepper to taste
- 1 teaspoon of butter or olive oil (optional)

Instructions:

- Crack the eggs into a bowl and whisk them thoroughly until well combined.
- Heat a non-stick skillet over medium-low heat. If using butter or oil, add it to the skillet.

- Pour the beaten eggs into the skillet and let them cook undisturbed for a minute or so until they start to set around the edges.
- Gently stir the eggs with a spatula, scraping from the edges to the center, until they are cooked through but still soft and slightly creamy.
- Season with salt and pepper to taste and serve warm.

Note: You can add chopped herbs like chives or parsley for extra flavor if tolerated.

2. Creamy Oatmeal with Applesauce

Ingredients:

- 1/2 cup rolled oats

- 1 cup water or milk (use lactose-free or almond milk if dairy is not tolerated)
- 1/4 cup unsweetened applesauce
- 1 tablespoon honey or maple syrup (optional)
- Dash of cinnamon (optional)

Instructions:

- In a small saucepan, bring the water or milk to a boil.
- Stir in the rolled oats and reduce the heat to low. Cook, stirring occasionally, until the oats are soft and creamy, about 5-7 minutes.
- Remove from heat and stir in the applesauce.
- Sweeten with honey or maple syrup if desired, and sprinkle with cinnamon.

- Serve warm.

3. Smoothie with Banana and Spinach

Ingredients:

- 1 ripe banana
- 1 cup fresh spinach leaves
- 1/2 cup plain yogurt (use lactose-free or almond milk yogurt if dairy is not tolerated)
- 1/2 cup water or almond milk
- 1 tablespoon honey or maple syrup (optional)

Instructions:

- Peel the banana and break it into chunks.
- Place the banana chunks, spinach leaves, yogurt, and water or almond milk in a blender.
- Blend until smooth and creamy.

- Sweeten with honey or maple syrup if desired.
- Pour into a glass and serve immediately.

Tips for Gastroparesis-Friendly Breakfasts:

- **Chew Thoroughly:** Even for soft foods like scrambled eggs or oatmeal, chewing well can aid digestion.
- **Small Portions:** Start with smaller portions and gradually increase as tolerated.
- **Hydration:** Drink fluids like water or herbal tea between meals to stay hydrated.

These breakfast recipes are designed to be gentle on the stomach while providing essential nutrients and energy to start your day. Adjust ingredients and portion sizes based on your individual tolerance and preferences.

Lunch Recipes

Here are a few lunch recipes that are suitable for individuals managing gastroparesis. These recipes focus on foods that are gentle on the stomach and easy to digest:

1. Chicken and Rice Soup

Ingredients:

- 1 boneless, skinless chicken breast, cut into small pieces
- 1 carrot, peeled and diced
- 1 celery stalk, diced
- 1/2 cup white rice
- 4 cups chicken broth (low-sodium if possible)

- Salt and pepper to taste

Instructions:

- In a large pot, bring the chicken broth to a boil.
- Add the diced chicken breast, carrot, celery, and white rice to the pot.
- Reduce heat to medium-low and simmer until the chicken is cooked through and the vegetables are tender, about 20 minutes.
- Season with salt and pepper to taste.
- Serve warm.

Note: You can puree the soup for a smoother texture if needed.

2. Quinoa Salad with Vegetables

Ingredients:

- 1 cup quinoa, rinsed
- 2 cups water or vegetable broth
- 1 cucumber, diced
- 1 bell pepper (any color), diced
- 1/4 cup chopped fresh parsley
- Juice of 1 lemon
- 2 tablespoons olive oil
- Salt and pepper to taste

Instructions:

- In a medium saucepan, bring the water or vegetable broth to a boil.
- Add the quinoa, reduce heat to low, cover, and simmer until quinoa is cooked and water is absorbed, about 15-20 minutes.

- Fluff the quinoa with a fork and let it cool to room temperature.
- In a large bowl, combine the cooked quinoa, diced cucumber, diced bell pepper, and chopped parsley.
- Drizzle with lemon juice and olive oil, and season with salt and pepper to taste.
- Toss gently to combine and serve chilled or at room temperature.

3. Tomato Basil Soup

Ingredients:

- 2 tablespoons olive oil
- 1 onion, diced
- 2 garlic cloves, minced
- 2 cans (14 oz each) diced tomatoes
- 2 cups vegetable broth (low-sodium if possible)

- 1/4 cup chopped fresh basil leaves
- Salt and pepper to taste

Instructions:

- Heat olive oil in a large pot over medium heat. Add diced onion and minced garlic, sauté until softened, about 5 minutes.
- Add diced tomatoes (with their juices) and vegetable broth to the pot. Bring to a boil, then reduce heat and simmer for 15-20 minutes.
- Remove from heat and stir in chopped fresh basil.
- Using an immersion blender or regular blender, puree the soup until smooth.
- Season with salt and pepper to taste.

- Serve warm, garnished with additional basil if desired.

Tips for Gastroparesis-Friendly Lunches:

- **Small Portions:** Start with smaller portions and eat slowly.
- **Avoid Heavy Sauces:** Choose recipes with light dressings or broths to avoid overwhelming the stomach.
- **Chew Thoroughly:** Even for soups or pureed dishes, chewing helps with digestion.

These lunch recipes provide nutritious options that are gentle on the stomach and can help manage symptoms of gastroparesis. Adjust ingredients and seasoning based on your individual tolerance and preferences.

Dinner Recipes

Here are some dinner recipes that are gentle on the stomach and suitable for individuals managing gastroparesis:

1. Baked Salmon with Lemon and Dill

Ingredients:

- 2 salmon fillets
- 1 lemon, sliced
- Fresh dill, chopped
- Salt and pepper to taste

Instructions:

- Preheat your oven to 375°F (190°C).
- Place the salmon fillets on a baking sheet lined with parchment paper.
- Season the salmon with salt and pepper to taste.

- Top each fillet with slices of lemon and sprinkle with chopped fresh dill.
- Bake in the preheated oven for 15-20 minutes, or until the salmon is cooked through and flakes easily with a fork.
- Serve warm with a side of mashed potatoes or steamed vegetables.

2. Turkey Meatballs in Marinara Sauce

Ingredients:

- 1 pound ground turkey
- 1/4 cup breadcrumbs
- 1 egg
- 1 teaspoon dried oregano
- Salt and pepper to taste
- 1 jar (16 oz) marinara sauce (low-sodium if possible)

Instructions:

- Preheat your oven to 375°F (190°C).
- In a mixing bowl, combine ground turkey, breadcrumbs, egg, dried oregano, salt, and pepper. Mix until well combined.
- Shape the mixture into meatballs and place them on a baking sheet lined with parchment paper.
- Bake in the preheated oven for 20-25 minutes, or until the meatballs are cooked through.
- In a saucepan, heat the marinara sauce over medium heat until warmed through.
- Serve the turkey meatballs with marinara sauce over soft-cooked pasta or rice.

3. Soft Tofu Stir-Fry with Vegetables

Ingredients:

- 1 block (14 oz) soft tofu, cut into cubes
- 1 cup sliced mushrooms
- 1 bell pepper (any color), sliced
- 1 cup snow peas
- 2 tablespoons soy sauce (low-sodium if possible)
- 1 tablespoon sesame oil
- 1 garlic clove, minced
- Salt and pepper to taste

Instructions:

- Heat sesame oil in a large skillet or wok over medium heat.
- Add minced garlic and sauté for 1-2 minutes, until fragrant.

- Add sliced mushrooms, bell pepper, and snow peas to the skillet. Stir-fry for 5-7 minutes, or until vegetables are tender-crisp.
- Add cubed tofu to the skillet and gently stir to combine with the vegetables.
- Drizzle soy sauce over the tofu and vegetables, and toss gently to coat.
- Season with salt and pepper to taste.
- Serve warm over white rice or quinoa.

Tips for Gastroparesis-Friendly Dinners:

• **Choose Soft Textures:** Opt for recipes that include soft-cooked or easily digestible ingredients like fish, tofu, and well-cooked vegetables.

- **Light Seasoning:** Use herbs, citrus, and mild spices for flavor without overwhelming the stomach.

- **Avoid Heavy Sauces:** Keep sauces light and use sparingly to avoid triggering symptoms.

These dinner recipes provide nutritious options that are gentle on the stomach and can help manage symptoms of gastroparesis. Adjust ingredients and seasoning based on your individual tolerance and preferences.

Snacks & Desserts Recipes

Here are some snack and dessert recipes that are gentle on the stomach and suitable for individuals managing gastroparesis:

Snack Recipes:

1. Smoothie with Banana and Spinach

Ingredients:

- 1 ripe banana
- 1 cup fresh spinach leaves
- 1/2 cup plain yogurt (use lactose-free or almond milk yogurt if dairy is not tolerated)
- 1/2 cup water or almond milk
- 1 tablespoon honey or maple syrup (optional)

Instructions:

- Peel the banana and break it into chunks.
- Place the banana chunks, spinach leaves, yogurt, and water or almond milk in a blender.
- Blend until smooth and creamy.
- Sweeten with honey or maple syrup if desired.
- Pour into a glass and serve immediately.

2. Applesauce with Cinnamon

Ingredients:

- 1 cup unsweetened applesauce
- Dash of cinnamon

Instructions:

- Spoon unsweetened applesauce into a small bowl.
- Sprinkle with a dash of cinnamon.
- Stir to combine.
- Serve chilled.

Dessert Recipes:

1. Rice Pudding

Ingredients:

- 1/2 cup white rice
- 2 cups milk (use lactose-free or almond milk if dairy is not tolerated)
- 1/4 cup sugar
- 1/2 teaspoon vanilla extract
- Dash of cinnamon

Instructions:

- In a medium saucepan, combine the rice and milk.
- Bring to a boil over medium heat, stirring occasionally.
- Reduce heat to low, cover, and simmer for 20-25 minutes, stirring occasionally, until rice is tender and mixture is creamy.
- Stir in sugar, vanilla extract, and cinnamon.
- Cook for an additional 5 minutes, stirring occasionally.
- Remove from heat and let cool slightly before serving warm or chilled.

2. Banana Yogurt Parfait

Ingredients:

- 1 ripe banana, sliced
- 1/2 cup plain yogurt (use lactose-free or almond milk yogurt if dairy is not tolerated)
- 2 tablespoons granola or crushed soft cookies (optional)

Instructions:

- In a small glass or bowl, layer sliced banana, yogurt, and granola or crushed soft cookies if using.
- Repeat layers until ingredients are used up.
- Serve immediately.

Tips for Gastroparesis-Friendly Snacks and Desserts:

- **Small Portions:** Start with smaller portions and eat slowly to avoid overwhelming the stomach.
- **Choose Soft Textures:** Opt for foods that are easy to chew and digest, like yogurt, applesauce, and smoothies.
- **Avoid Heavy Sugars and Fats:** Use natural sweeteners like honey or maple syrup sparingly, and opt for low-fat or non-fat options when possible.

These snack and dessert recipes provide nutritious options that are gentle on the stomach and can help manage symptoms of gastroparesis.

Adjust ingredients and portion sizes based on your individual tolerance and preferences.

CHAPTER FOUR
Coping With Gastroparesis Symptoms

Coping with gastroparesis symptoms involves a combination of lifestyle adjustments, dietary changes, medical treatments, and coping strategies to manage the condition effectively. Here are some tips to help cope with gastroparesis symptoms:

1. Dietary Adjustments:

- **Small, Frequent Meals:** Eat smaller meals throughout the day to reduce the workload on your digestive system.
- **Soft and Well-Cooked Foods:** Opt for foods that are easier to digest, such as steamed vegetables, tender meats, and cooked grains.

- **Low-Fat and Low-Fiber Choices:** Limit high-fat and high-fiber foods that can delay gastric emptying and exacerbate symptoms.
- **Fluids and Hydration:** Stay hydrated by sipping fluids between meals, but avoid large amounts of liquid at once.
- **Identify Trigger Foods:** Keep a food diary to identify and avoid foods that worsen your symptoms.

2. Meal Planning:

- Plan meals and snacks ahead of time to ensure you have gastroparesis-friendly options available.
- Work with a registered dietitian to create a personalized meal plan

that meets your nutritional needs and helps manage symptoms.

3. Medications and Treatments:

- Follow your healthcare provider's recommendations regarding medications to help manage symptoms such as nausea, vomiting, and abdominal pain.
- Consider medications that promote stomach emptying (prokinetics) or control symptoms (antiemetics).

4. Lifestyle Adjustments:

- **Physical Activity:** Engage in light physical activity, such as walking, to promote digestion and overall well-being.

- **Stress Management:** Practice stress-reducing techniques such as deep breathing, meditation, or yoga, as stress can exacerbate symptoms.

5. Supportive Therapies:

- **Acupuncture:** Some individuals find relief from gastroparesis symptoms through acupuncture.
- **Biofeedback:** This technique can help train the muscles involved in digestion and improve symptoms.

Understand that managing gastroparesis can be a journey of trial and adjustment. Be patient with yourself and persistent in finding what works best for managing your symptoms.

Symptoms of gastroparesis can be effectively managed and your quality of life can be enhanced by collaborating with your healthcare team and implementing these coping strategies. It is crucial to identify a personalized approach that is appropriate for your specific requirements, as the experience of gastroparesis may differ from person to person.

Conclusion

A multifaceted approach to managing gastroparesis is necessary, which includes dietary adjustments, lifestyle modifications, medical remedies, and coping strategies. This chronic condition impairs digestion by delaying or obstructing the stomach's proper evacuation, resulting in symptoms such as bloating, nausea, and discomfort.

Key aspects of managing gastroparesis include:

- **Dietary Modifications:** Choosing foods that are easy to digest, low in fat and fiber, and consuming small, frequent meals can help alleviate symptoms and improve digestion.

- **Medications and Treatments:** Working with healthcare providers to explore medications that promote stomach emptying (prokinetics) or control symptoms (antiemetics) is crucial.

- **Lifestyle Adjustments:** Incorporating light physical activity, stress management techniques, and regular medical monitoring can contribute to overall symptom management and well-being.

- **Support and Education:** Seeking support from healthcare professionals, joining support groups, and staying informed about gastroparesis can provide valuable resources and emotional support.

- **Personalized Care:** Each individual may respond differently to treatments and dietary changes, so a personalized approach tailored to specific symptoms and needs is essential.

Individuals can enhance their quality of life and effectively manage gastroparesis by adhering to these strategies and maintaining open communication with healthcare providers. Although gastroparesis presents challenges, proactive management and adaptation can enable individuals to lead fulfilling lives while reducing the severity of symptoms.

THE END

www.ingramcontent.com/pod-product-compliance
Lightning Source LLC
Chambersburg PA
CBHW070207230526
45471CB00002B/864